Crikey I'm...

A Mum

Other titles in the *Crikey I'm...* series

Crikey I'm A Teenager
Crikey I'm Thirty
Crikey I'm Forty
Crikey I'm Fifty
Crikey I'm Retired
Crikey I'm Getting Married
Crikey I'm In Love
Crikey I'm A Dad
Crikey I'm A Grandparent

Crikey I'm... A Mum

Contributors

**Dr David Haslam
Victoria Warner
Eliza Williams**

Edited by

Steve Hare

Cover Illustration by

Ian Pollock

PURPLE HOUSE

Published by Purple House Limited 1998
75 Banbury Road
Oxford OX2 6PE

© Purple House Limited 1998

Cover illustration: © Ian Pollock/The Inkshed

Crikey I'm... is a trademark of Purple House Limited

A catalogue record for this book is available from the British Library

ISBN 1-84118-016-5

All rights reserved. No part of this publication may be reproduced, stored in a retrieval system, or transmitted, in any form or by any means, electronic, mechanical, photocopying, recording or otherwise, without the prior permission of the publishers.

Printed in Great Britain by
Cox and Wyman

Acknowledgements

We are grateful to everyone who helped in the compilation of this book, particularly to the following:

Stephen Franks of Franks and Franks (Design)

Inform Group Worldwide (Reproduction)

Dave Kent of the Kobal Collection

Parents at Work

Bodleian Library, Oxford

Central Library, Oxford

British Film Institute

National Office of Statistics

Liz Brown

Eric and Amy Guttensohn

Mark McClintock

Hannah Wren

Illustrations

The Fugitive	3
A Ladybird book	4
A 1971 Cow & Gate advertisement	8
A Private Affair	10
Nurse Harvey's Gripe Water	12
Lorenzo Di Credi's *Virgin and Child*	15
The Lady is Willing	18
A 1986 advertisement for Oxo	21
Sparrows	25
A 1998 Britvic advertisement	29
Dr Spock's *Baby and Child Care*	30
The Guttensohn Quintuplets	34
A 1957 Johnson & Johnson advertisement	38
Domestic bliss from an early film	42
A 1972 Lucozade advertisement	47
Simon Vouet's *Virgin and Child*	48

Contents

Crikey I'm A Mum!   **1**

Mother Care   **5**

Hard Labour   **17**

Keeping Abreast of Tradition   **22**

The Morning After   **24**

Labour Intensive   **28**

A Fit Mum   **31**

Magical Mothers   **39**

Thank You for Having Me   **49**

Crikey, I'm A Mum!

It's the biggest event in your life so far: you're a mother. Months of waiting and anticipation have led up to this moment, when you hold that precious bundle in your arms for the first time – the beginning of a new life which will change yours forever.

Understandably, your feelings are mixed. You've been waiting so long for a glimpse of your child, to hold it in your arms, to touch it and embrace it with that legendary maternal love. On the other hand, the responsibility seems overwhelming: you're going to be in charge of a new life, and for the next 18 years – and the rest – it (or they) will depend on you for food, clothing, love and almost every other aspect of life. And the baby seems so small, fragile and helpless: what if you break it?

On the other hand, you know that having a baby is the nearest thing there is to a miracle. You have created a new life; your place in the grand scheme of things is assured; you have made contact with eternity.

Being a mum means so many different things to different people. These days becoming a mother doesn't necessarily entail giving up work; nor does it mean that you have to maintain a career simultaneously. Advice is everywhere – everybody's got something to say about how to bring up, and bond with, your baby. But what about you, the mother? Where does the mum herself fit into all of this?

Regardless of how you're looking at it, motherhood marks the greatest landmark in your existence so far; the most significant stage in any woman's life. After all, in biological terms, reproduction is the sole point of our existence. You're being admitted to a very special and deeply personal club: no one can possibly even begin to imagine being a mum until they actually become one. Hidden beneath the piles of dirty nappies, at the bottom of all the feeding bottles, and at the heart of all those sticky hugs is the idea of motherhood – and that alone makes everything worthwhile.

Congratulations, Mum. Everything about you should be celebrated – past, present, future, body, mind and soul; so put the baby clothes down, put your feet up, and enjoy to the full this exhilarating new experience.

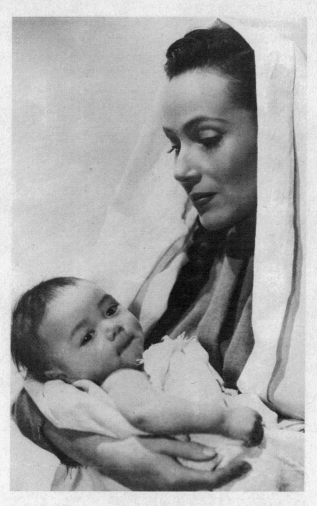

A serene maternal moment in *The Fugitive*, 1947.

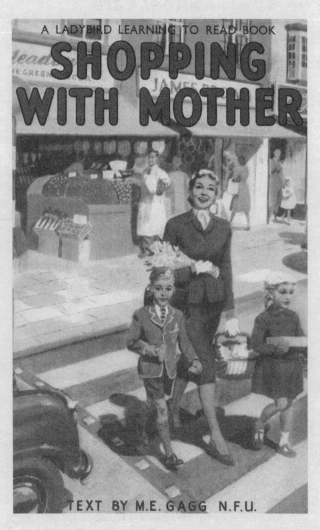

A classic Ladybird book, first published in 1958.

Mother Care

A History of Motherhood

There must have been a time in our ancient past when the sex act and the birth of a baby some nine months later were viewed as quite separate and unrelated occurrences. People walked, sat, ate, defecated, killed, had sex and had babies. One act did not cause the other. Plants died and new ones appeared in the spring. Animals and birds had young. The sun rose each morning and died again each night. Miracles happened.

In primitive times the life expectancy of men and women was not great: surviving to their mid thirties was a real achievement. But then, unlike today, it was the men who lived longer. Men might face the daily dangers of wild animals, marauding raiders and battle; but women had the rigours and real dangers of recurrent childbirth to contend with.

In the earliest cultures, where the nuclear family was unknown, women possessed a power and status in their societies that they have only begun to win back this century. There could only ever be certainty about the mother of any child; the father could be any of the males with whom she associated.

> ### Matronalia
>
> Matronalia was the festival of Juno on 1 March, when prayers were offered to her and to her son Mars. It was also the old New Year's Day, when women served food to slaves and married ladies received presents from married men.

And it was the mother, caring for her children, who possessed the power of life or death over those children and thus the success and survival of the group to which she belonged. The earliest gods were women, with goddesses representing motherhood and the miracle of regeneration.

Raising children was in itself a full-time occupation, with agriculture, animal husbandry and cooking no doubt thrown in for good measure. And the constant round of pregnancy, birth and care would inevitably take its toll. The men might be broken, but the women just wore out.

> Women are having children later and having fewer of them. By the age of 30, women born in 1936 had an average of 1.9 children compared with only 1.3 children to women born in 1966.

By the time history came to be recorded in writing, rather than through surviving artefacts and cave paintings, society, in just about every country, was organised around men, and women were relegated to an inferior status, often only one step above actual slavery. The most powerful gods had all become male, too.

The Bible has a great deal to say on the subject, and though the New Testament is considerably more relaxed than the Old, it can still be a little hard to take literally at the end of the twentieth century: 'Wives, submit yourselves unto your own husbands, as unto the Lord. For the husband is the head of the wife, even as Christ is the head of the church: and he is the saviour of the body' (Ephesians 5:22–33).

It had been taught for generations that labour pains had originally been inflicted on women because of the sin of Eve in the Garden of Eden. The Fall was Eve's fault, and Adam was not slow to pass on this information, and got off rather lightly in consequence. 'I will greatly multiply thy sorrow and thy conception,' it says in Genesis, 'in sorrow thou shalt bring forth children; and thy desire shall be to thy husband, and he shall rule over you.' The creation of Eve herself, of course, was depicted – possibly because of a mistranslation – as an afterthought, fashioned from a spare part of Adam.

> 'Children seldom misquote you. In fact, they usually repeat word for word what you shouldn't have said.'
> Anon.

Women in medieval Britain would typically spend the great majority of their adult lives being reminded of Eve's fallibility, bearing and rearing children, often on an almost annual basis. The ideal of a good woman was, not unnaturally, inextricably linked with motherhood. On the other hand, in the case of a childless marriage, it was always assumed that the fault must lie with the mother.

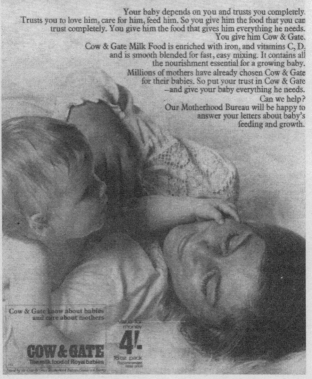

Bonding with Cow & Gate in 1971.

> **Under the Skin**
>
> After a 17th-century birth, women were wrapped in the skin of a sheep. If a sheep wasn't available, a hare would do – although presumably more than one was needed!

While contraception was either non-existent or based on a fairly rudimentary knowledge of human anatomy and reproduction (it was once held that red-headed children were the result of conception during menstruation), a natural form operated, based, conveniently, on wealth. Ladies of society and from wealthy families would put out new-born children to a wet-nurse. The act of breast-feeding would tend to lessen the risk of pregnancy among poorer families. The wealthy woman of leisure, on the other hand, would soon be back to normal. Otherwise, there was a vast store of gossip and rumour and the products of quacks or witches to procure abortions for those already overburdened with children, or for whom a pregnancy was inconvenient. The potions were often fatal to both.

Pregnancy was generally regarded as a period of ill-health. Women were advised not to travel in carriages or ride on the dreadful roads that existed, or take any strenuous exercise. Giving birth was a risky business,

> The rate of multiple births in the UK rose over the last decade from 10.8 per thousand maternities in 1986 to 13.8 in 1996.

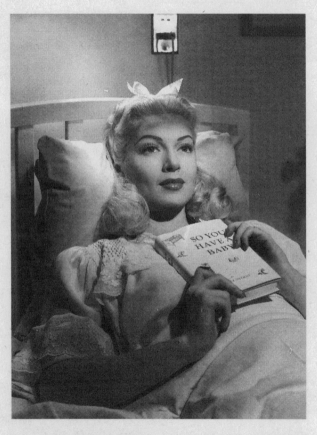

Lana Turner recovers quickly from childbirth in *Marriage is a Private Affair*, 1944.

which increased with every child born. Complications which are almost routine matters today were commonly fatal until the last century, when surgical techniques were refined and reliable anaesthetics became available. So pregnancy was always a cause for concern. Even after a successful birth, the risks were not over, and a substantial percentage of children – at times around 20 per cent of all born – failed to survive infancy.

Before the nineteenth century, most improvements in the health of mothers and their infants were more accidental than scientific. It is recorded, for instance, that the introduction of iron cooking pots significantly helped reduce the incidence of anaemia. Otherwise, wives and husbands depended on hearsay and guesswork, or the bizarre *Aristotle's Masterpiece*, first published in Britain in the seventeenth century and still in use earlier this century, despite the fact that it talked of 'phlegm', 'humours' and 'monstrous births', and suggested that a baby with a hare-lip could only be the result of the mother meeting a hare while pregnant.

Unlocking the Past

It was once traditional, on the island of Salsette near Bombay, to open all the locks of doors and drawers, in order to make labour easier for the pregnant woman.

Only the most desperate and unlucky mothers gave birth alone. The majority would be attended at the

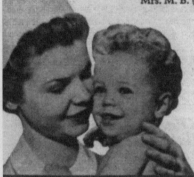

Nurse Harvey gives advice to fifties mums.

very least by a friend or neighbour. Traditionally, the husband would be nearby but not present. Many were attended by experienced midwives, though it must be said that an important part of the midwife's training was to administer baptism to any child unlikely to survive. It was widely believed that unbaptised children could not enter the kingdom of Heaven. If the mother died before the birth, the baby might be removed from the womb to be buried separately. Early midwives were often regarded as not that much different from witches. In 1591 a midwife was burnt at the stake for administering an opiate painkiller to a woman in labour.

Children did not necessarily stay at home or even near when they started to work, which could be at almost any age after infancy. It was common for them to be separated by some distance, only returning for special celebrations and holidays. The more wealthy parents might send their child to a monastery to learn the basic subjects and Latin.

The introduction of chloroform in the nineteenth century meant privileged women could, once again, lie back and

> Lone parents headed around 21% of all families with dependent children in Britain in 1996, which was nearly three times the proportion in 1971, although the rate of increase may have slowed recently. Most lone-parent families are headed by a lone mother.

> ### Fruitful and Fertile
>
> **Thinking of trying for another? According to Aristotle, to promote fertility a woman should:**
>
> *'make a suffumigation of red styrax, myrrh, cassia-wood, nutmeg, and cinnamon, and let her receive the fumes into her womb, covering her very close; and if the odour so received passes through the body to the mouth and nostrils, she is fruitful.'*

think of England, and play no active part in the most important moment of their lives. Yet even in the 1920s it was pointed out, to great effect, that it was four times more dangerous to bear a child than to work in a mine.

The move away from home births to hospitals began in earnest. The introduction of the National Health Service after World War Two, along with the availability of antibiotics, vitamins and free orange juice for infants rapidly reduced the risks of childbirth and infant mortality. And the growing acceptance of the necessity for contraception – officially endorsed by the Church of England in 1958, meant that parenthood could finally be a matter of choice, rather than chance. The introduction of the contraceptive pill in the 1960s was initially greeted as the perfect solution – as much by liberated women as by carefree men.

Throughout the great majority of history, with few exceptions, right until the latter half of this century, childbirth has been viewed as the exclusive province

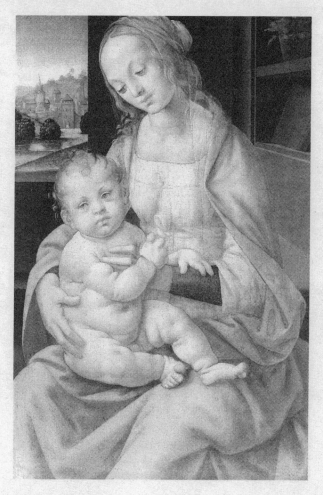

Virgin and Child, Lorenzo di Credi, c. 1485; Ashmolean Museum, Oxford.

of women. Films and TV dramas in the 1960s still portrayed the father nervously pacing the waiting-room floor, chain-smoking, and later distributing cigars in his local. Today's new man, of course, is fully involved – and has eschewed all forms of smoking long since.

Average Births per Woman Across the World

UK 1.8	Hong Kong 1.2
Afghanistan 6.9	Laos 6.7
Belize 4.2	Malawi 7.2
Cameroon 5.7	Malaysia 3.6
Austria 1.5	Oman 7.2
China 2.0	Rwanda 6.6
Congo 6.3	Somalia 7.0
Gambia 5.6	Spain 1.2
Germany 1.3	Thailand 2.1
Uganda 7.3	Yemen 7.6

Hard Labour

British Traditions of Birth

So you think birth is complicated now? You should have been alive a couple of hundred years ago. Back then, women didn't have any kind of choice about where or how they gave birth: no one could choose between hospital and home, because hospitals simply didn't cater for that kind of thing. Home it was then, usually in a room especially put aside for this purpose: but the whole process of childbirth certainly involved much more than the actual labour, and could go on for a whole month in total.

> **Wetting the Baby's Head**
>
> In past centuries, mothers who had just given birth were given a special drink called caudle: it consisted of ale and wine, warmed with sugar and spices; probably just what they needed after a long, hard labour.

Until around the turn of the last century, it was Christianity and the Bible which had provided guidelines for women giving birth in English society. The rules were clear, rigid, and centuries-old.

When the time for birth came, the pregnant woman was always surrounded by a group of other female friends. They were the 'gossips': the meaning of the word comes from 'God-sib' or 'God-sibling'. These women were there specifically to witness the birth, their testimony being necessary at the baptism later.

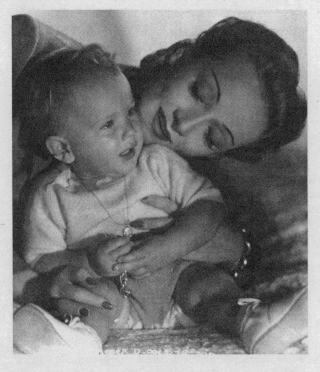

Marlene Dietrich adopts a baby in *The Lady is Willing*, 1942.

> **'The first half of our lives is ruined by our parents, and the second half by our children.'**
>
> Clarence Darrow

When the actual birth was finally over, the woman was still considered to be 'unclean'. In England, the origin of this idea comes from Leviticus Chapter 12, which says that a woman is 'impure' for 40 days after the birth of a baby boy; and 80 after the birth of a baby girl.

The new mother, then, had to resign herself simply to not stirring from the house for a month or so. After five days the bed linen was changed – not before time, one imagines – and after that the mother could move about the room (this momentous event was called upsitting).

With the month finally up, there was only one ritual left for the new mother: churching. This was a rite of purification, and it basically admitted the mother back into society, involving a blessing and a special service. We are left, though, with one small question: if the mother couldn't go outside until she was churched, how did she get to the church in the first place? History is a strange thing.

Who Will It Resemble?

What will the baby look like? Back in the seventeenth century, it was much easier to tell. Apparently, the appearance of the baby depended entirely on what the mother was thinking about, both during the 'act' of conception, and also the pregnancy itself.

For example, if the mother were 'copulating unlawfully' with a lover, and she thought of her husband, the child conceived would resemble the husband rather than its natural father. If the mother even looks closely at an object, the child would be born with the mark of that object somewhere upon its body: probably in the shape of a birthmark or mole.

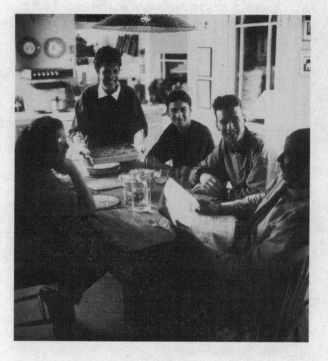

Happy families – Lynda Bellingham and the Oxo clan in 1985.

Keeping Abreast of Tradition

Breast-feeding Through the Centuries

These days, the decision to breast-feed your baby is yours alone. Hundreds of years ago, however, things were rather different: not only should the child be breast-fed (either by you or by someone else), but people had rather strange ideas about the whole process...

- In the Middle Ages, many 'experts' believed that breast milk was actually menstrual blood which had been heated and whitened by the heat of the mother's body.

- Right up until the last century, most people believed that breast-feeding mothers should in no way become 'over-excited'. 'Passionate excitement' on the part of the mother would lead to convulsions in the child which 'could be fatal', according to a nineteenth-century 'mothers' manual'.

> 'A wet-nurse should neither be too young nor too old; not more than 30, nor less than 20 years of age; of a good constitution, and not suffering under, or especially liable to, any complaint... She should be good-tempered, and not subject to fits of passion.'
>
> From *The Marriage Almanack and Mother's Manual*, 183

Left Holding the Baby

If you were an upper-class mother in a previous century, there's little chance that you would actually have breast-fed the baby yourself: you'd have hired, instead, a wet-nurse. This woman would have had a child recently herself, and her sole purpose was to breast-feed your baby, thus giving it the best possible start in life. With another woman feeding your child, you of course would have been able to get pregnant yet again in a relatively short time.

Once feeding your child, the wet-nurse had to prioritise it, in every way, above her own. There is an unhappy episode in Dickens's novel *Dombey and Son* where the wet-nurse, Toodles, is forced to leave her whole family, including her new baby, behind, in order for her to devote herself uninterruptedly to Mr Dombey's delicate young son. Such occasions, Dickens would have us believe, were far from rare and were exceedingly traumatic for all involved.

The Morning After

Maternity Around The World

The idea of new mothers being 'unclean' exists more or less around the world, and is very ancient. Indeed, many cultures, both primitive and modern, still consider the woman to be impure for a certain number of days after the birth, although the actual length of this time varies.

In Sikh tradition, women are not allowed to prepare food for 40 days after the birth (an opportunity any woman should perhaps make the most of). Hindu new mothers are similarly considered to be 'unclean', although the length of time for this varies according to their caste. For a high-caste Brahmin, for example, the period lasts for 10 days; but for a low-caste Sudra, it is 30 days. At the end of this, the mother is expected to take a purifying bath.

Male Protection

To assist with easy delivery, in the Philippines, the husband would stand stark naked in the hut with a drawn sword to ward off spirits.

A new Jewish mother is looked after very carefully: childbirth is seen as a potentially life-threatening situation, and the pregnancy can be terminated at any point before the child's head has been delivered, if the mother's life is in danger. After this, the child is a separate human being, whose life cannot be sacrificed, even if the mother is in danger herself. Following the birth, a

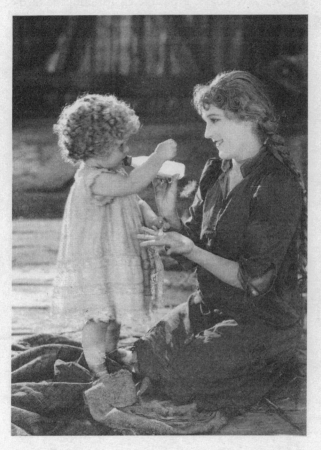

Mary Pickford in a tender moment from *Sparrows*, 1926.

mother is traditionally excused from any fasting for the first seven days. From the eighth until the thirtieth day, she must fast only during Yom Kippur – and then only if she is thoroughly healthy.

A few cultures were more worried about the vulnerability of the mother than about her ability to pollute everything. In Greece, for example, it was traditionally believed that women in labour were susceptible to the evil eye, and all mirrors were removed from the room (on the rather bizarre pretext that it was possible to put the evil eye on yourself). In primitive societies, knots were considered to be harbingers of evil, and so all knots were untied to help the mother relax. It was generally believed that any tied knots would similarly 'tie up' the mother, and obstruct the birth. The idea, basically, was that everything should be allowed to 'flow freely', and that would encourage a healthy birth.

As a further precaution, doors and windows were sometimes bolted to keep out evil spirits. In India, mothers felt safe by hiding a weapon under the bed as protection against evil spirits.

After the Birth

In *Java*, the afterbirth is given to the crocodiles to eat, as the souls of the forefathers live in these animals.

Among the *Swahili*, the placenta is buried on the spot where the birth took place. The cord should be wound round the child's neck for some time – presumably until it shrivelled up.

In *Spain*, it was once held that if the afterbirth is eaten by an animal, the child will acquire the bad habits of that animal.

In *Kwakiutl*, of British Columbia, the afterbirth of a baby boy was given to a raven to eat, giving the boy the power of foretelling the future; a girl's was buried at high tide mark, so that she would become an expert clam-digger.

The custom of planting a tree over the buried afterbirth is intended to mirror the child's own development.

Labour Intensive

Couvade Customs

While tradition throughout history has generally dictated that fathers suffer enforced absence while their wives gave birth, the experience might still be shared in different ways. Couvade was a common custom whereby the husband simulated labour and the birth of his child. This might involve simply going to bed, or actually experiencing the pains of sympathetic labour. Such customs were still practised earlier this century. There are various theories as to the purpose of couvade. In a rather less organised society it might be a formal means of demonstrating or asserting paternity. Or, as was common with many rituals and customs, it might have originated as a ploy to distract the evil spirits who might otherwise have attacked his wife and child at this vulnerable time.

The nineteenth-century anthropologist Sir Everard im Thurn gave this bizarre account of couvade in British Guyana:

> Even before the child is born, the father abstains for a time from certain kinds of animal food. The woman works as usual up to a few hours before the birth of the child. At last she retires alone, or accompanied by some other women, to the forest, where she ties up her hammock; and then the child is born. Then, in a few hours – often less than a day – the woman, who like all women living in a very unartificial condition, suffers but little, gets up

and resumes her ordinary work. In any case, no sooner is the child born than the father takes to his hammock, and, abstaining from every sort of work, from meat and all other food, except weak gruel of cassava meal, from smoking, from washing himself, and, above all, from touching weapons of any sort, is nursed and cared for by all the women of the place. One other regulation is certainly quaint: the interesting father may not scratch himself with his finger-nails, but he may use for this purpose a splinter, specially provided, from the mid-rib of a cokerite palm. This continues for many days and sometimes even weeks.

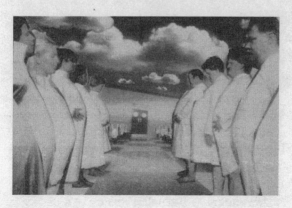

Men and women share the joys of pregnancy in this 1998 Britvic advertisement.

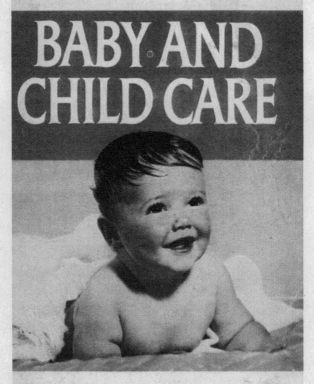

The seminal fifties baby care book, first published in 1946.

A Fit Mum

Dr David Haslam

It's wonderful, and it's terrifying. Few moments in life are quite as thrilling and world-changing as becoming a parent. No matter how much you may have read about parenthood, or however many ante-natal classes you went to, nothing can completely prepare you for the real thing. When you first held your baby in your arms, you were probably filled with a mixture of overwhelming love, bewilderment, a realisation of the enormity of the responsibility ahead, and not a little exhaustion!

Being a mum will give you the highest highs, but will also bring more than its fair share of anxiety and worry. Having a baby changes absolutely everything, for ever. The level of responsibility that children bring is greater than anything you will have ever experienced before. There is no time off, no days when you are not a mum. That doesn't mean you will be always working – though it may feel like it to begin with. But it does mean that for both parents, life will never be the same again. And the great majority of you wouldn't want it any other way – most of the time.

Your Changing Body
- Don't be surprised if you feel physically exhausted to begin with. Tiredness is entirely to be expected in the first few weeks, especially if your baby repeatedly disturbs your sleep. If necessary, your GP will check that you are not anaemic when you have your

post-natal check.

- Many babies take quite a while to develop a 'civilised' sleep pattern, so grab your sleep when you can. If your baby sleeps after lunch, then you should, too.

- There is no doubt that there are benefits to both mother and baby from breast-feeding, but if you simply don't feel that this is for you after you have given it a try, then please don't feel guilty.

- Don't smoke. If you are still smoking, it is essential to stop now. Babies whose parents smoke have a higher incidence of many conditions, including asthma and ear infections; instances of cot death are also significantly higher. Can you possibly still smoke, knowing that? If you need help, talk to your doctor or practice nurse.

- Don't be alarmed if you don't go back to your pre-pregnancy weight straight away. Don't go on a slimming diet to begin with, but make sure you have plenty of high fibre foods, fruit and vegetables.

- After giving birth, your abdominal muscles will inevitably be rather flabby. They have been very stretched recently! So do work on the exercises you were taught, and practise pulling in your tummy muscles during odd moments when you are standing still.

- From a strictly medical point of view it is safe to resume sexual intercourse at about two weeks –

provided any discharge has stopped, and any stitches have healed. However, most couples wait very much longer than this. Even after any bruising and soreness has eased, sex drive is still definitely reduced in many women, which could be nature's way of spreading families out. Some partners feel resentful of this, particularly as so much of your attention is now directed towards the baby. So talk about it, explain how you feel, and stress that you still love and fancy him. In time, you will both feel ready for love-making to start again.

Your Changing Emotions

The job description of parenthood would probably read:

Hours: Limitless.

Time off: Virtually none – at least during the first five years in post.

Payment: Usually none.

Sick pay: None.

Training: Minimal.

Conditions: No legal controls.

Skills: Unlimited, but applicants should be willing to take on cooking, cleaning, washing, nursing, teaching, taxi-driving, first aid, ironing, blame-taking, and counselling.

Responsibilities: Enormous: the development of the next generation.

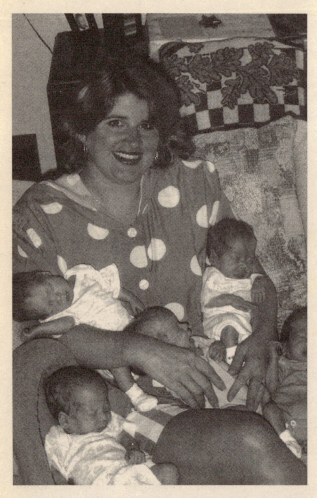

Amy Guttensohn of Montgomery, Alabama, proud mother of all-male quintuplets Taylor, Mason, Hunter, Parker and Tanner; born 8 August 1996.

Don't be surprised, then, if you find the job stressful at times. Don't bottle up your worries. Instead, do talk to other parents. It only seems that everyone else is finding it easier than you. In truth, they are probably finding it just as hard.

Don't worry if you don't feel overwhelming love for your new baby right from the start. Many mothers do feel guilty and worried that their feelings are not quite how they had expected, but in most cases the feelings deepen over the next weeks and months as your baby becomes more of an individual.

The 'baby blues' are almost universal, typically starting on the third or fourth day. But if you develop feelings of weepiness, panic, feel unable to cope, and have little interest in your baby, your partner, or your home, then you may be developing post-natal depression. This affects around five per cent of mothers, and no one is immune. It is very treatable, so contact your GP, midwife, or health visitor right away.

Don't be surprised if everyone who visits gives all their attention to the baby, and little to you; and don't be jealous. They do care about you.

At the start, there will seem to be an impossible number of tasks that all need doing. However, after the first few weeks you will develop a routine, and you will soon astonish yourself by changing nappies, bathing, and feeding your baby as if you had been doing it all your life. Your partner should be doing his share as well, though do try and avoid taking over and showing him how everything should be done, just because you've developed more expertise. It can be very dispiriting for him, and may even dampen his enthusiasm to help.

It may be a cliché, but you will soon discover that your children grow up quicker than you ever could have believed. So enjoy these times with them, and take lots of photographs. You will never be able to revisit past days, so capture as many as you can with your camera or video camera.

Becoming a mum will have changed your life for ever, but you also need to remember that you and your partner still need time together. Don't take each other for granted: something all too easy to do. Meanwhile, you can both enjoy the fact that your baby will look at you as if you are the most wonderful, beautiful, fascinating, safe and secure person that ever existed. For your baby, you are. It's a great feeling.

David Haslam is married with two children and has been a GP for 22 years. He is a Fellow of the Royal College of General Practitioners, and has written numerous books – the most recent being Stress Free Parenting. *He also writes a column for* Practical Parenting *magazine, and frequently broadcasts on health topics*

Mother

Ian Paisley said last week that the Stormont peace package was "the mother of all betrayals". I began to think that any moment the reverend was going to sprout an enormous black moustache. Where had we all heard that form of words before? Surely it was in 1991 when Saddam was looking forward to "the mother of all battles". (Mr Paisley had already said, almost complacently it seemed to me, that a peace deal in Ulster would lead to war.)

It seems rather hard that war, which is mostly a male activity, should be regarded as female. Yet "the father of all wars" doesn't have the same ring, and in any case means something different. Chaucer is called the father of English poetry and George Stephenson the father of railways, and the father of wars would be taken to be the person who invented warfare. Necessity is the mother of invention, it is true, but she is an abstraction, not a flesh-and-blood creature as Chaucer and Stephenson were.

When it comes to metaphors, mothers carry much more clout than fathers do, since they nourish life. Victorian etymologists said that "Mamma", the child's word for its mother in so many languages, was "a mere repetition of 'ma', an infantile syllable", as Walter Skeat put it, and the 1989 edition of the *OED* says the same ("A reduplicated syllable often uttered instinctively by young children"); and it is no coincidence that mamma is also the Latin for breast. I suppose the Romans chose it because their own children kept on repeating that "infantile syllable". Liddell and Scott say mamman was Greek for "to cry for the mother's breast". Anyway, "Mummy" and "Mum" are corruptions of mamma, not of the quite different mother.

From 'Words', by Nicholas Bagnall;
Independent On Sunday; 19 April 1998

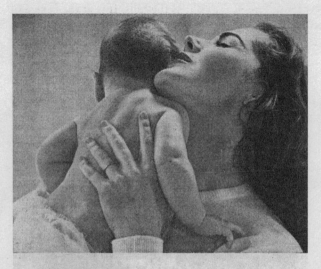

LOVING CARE...JOHNSON'S BABY CARE

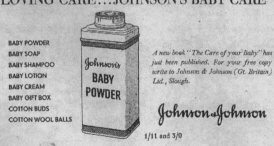

Johnson & Johnson provide a soft touch back in 1957 (with thanks to Johnson & Johnson).

Magical Mothers

Mum Myths and Legends

Motherhood is as old as the hills. It is at the centre of everybody's life – everybody has a mother, and mothers have been there since the very beginning of creation. It is not surprising, then, that thousands of myths and legends surround motherhood in all its many varied forms, from mythological mums, to the famous mothers of our own generation.

Persephone and Demeter

The Greek god of the Underworld, Pluto, was out in his chariot inspecting the foundations of Sicily. It was an unstable place, even in those days, not simply because of Mount Etna's occasional eruptions, but for the fact that the entire island was there to keep the giant Typhoeus pinned down, as punishment for some ancient rebellion against the gods.

The goddess of love, Aphrodite, was in a bad mood over some slight to her dignity. It occurred to her, seeing Pluto, that while the entire earth and all the oceans were slaves to the power of love, the Underworld was totally devoid of romance. She asked her son, Eros, to change all this by shooting one of his magic arrows into Pluto's heart, so that he would fall in love with Persephone, the daughter of Demeter.

> **733,300 babies were born in Great Britain in 1996.**

It worked. Pluto saw Persephone and was smitten instantly. Gods are not the sort of people to consider the normal courtesies in such matters. He just grabbed her and carried her off to his dark home.

Demeter was distraught. She searched the world in vain, and because her daughter was lost in Sicily, she took her revenge on that country. Demeter, Ceres to the Romans, was the goddess of growth: her name is the origin of our word, 'cereal', the edible grain of wheat, oats or barley. Ultimately, she vowed that nothing would grow in the world until her daughter was restored to her.

Eventually news reached Demeter that her daughter was in the Underworld. She took her case to Zeus, the

Fundamentalism

As you may well be finding out by now, piles can be the bane of any new mother's life. Now, however, you can put that rubber ring down and heave a huge sigh of relief: the 17th-century *Aristotle's Masterpiece*, the indispensable guide to all matters maternal and sexual, has the solution.

'Take an onion, and having made a hole in the middle of it, fill it full of oil, roast it, and having bruised it altogether, apply it to the fundament.'

Doesn't appeal? Try this alternative:

'Take a dozen of snails without shells, if you can get them [i.e. slugs], *or else so many shell snails, and pull them out, and having bruised them with a little oil, apply them warm as before* [i.e. to the bottom].'

king of all the gods – and, incidentally, Persephone's father – who ruled that she could return to the living world only if she had eaten nothing since her abduction. But she had: just seven seeds from a single pomegranate. The ultimate decision, therefore, was that she should be allowed to live in our world for a third of the year, and return to the Underworld for the other two-thirds.

Demeter, the mother of all things, forever rejoiced during those months when her precious daughter was returned to her, but mourned for the remaining months. Thus it was that the world acquired seasons. Prior to the abduction, the world endured perpetual spring; now we have to suffer the cold months of winter, in memory of the loss of the daughter of Demeter.

Inanna

Inanna was a legendary mother figure, the Sumerian goddess of fertility. She abandoned heaven and earth, and went down to the Underworld. After donning her ceremonial robes, Inanna instructed her vizier Ninshubur that if she didn't come back, he had to go to the god Enlil and ask for his help in rescuing her from the Underworld. Should he refuse, Ninshubur had to go to her father, the moon god, Nanna, with the same request. If he wouldn't help, Ninshubur had to approach Enki, the god of wisdom and sweet water. Inanna was admitted into the Underworld by Ereshkigal, her elderly sister. However, at each of the different seven gates of the Underworld, she was

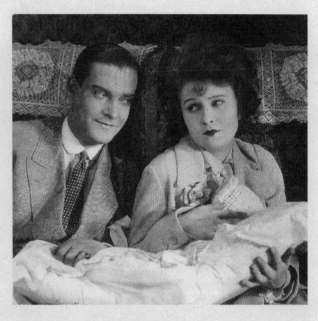

Happy families?

stripped of her robes, and when she arrived in front of her sister she was naked. She was killed by the gaze of the seven judges of the Underworld, and her body was hung upon a stake.

Meskhenet

Meskhenet was the goddess of childbirth in Ancient Egypt. She is shown as a woman with two loops over a vertical stroke, thought to be the bicornate uterus of a heifer, on her head. She ensures the safe delivery of the child by acting as a sacred midwife, and she affects the destiny of the child. Taweret is another goddess of childbirth: a hippopotamus goddess, with the head of a hippo, the limbs of a lion, the tail of a crocodile and large breasts. In Ancient Egypt, they used to make vases in her shape; when the milk was poured, it was poured through the nipples and gave the liquid a magic property.

Europa

Europa was playing in the fields one day when she was tricked by a beautiful white bull (Zeus in disguise). He allowed her to put flowers into his mouth, and she climbed onto his back. Eventually he carried her off to Crete, where Zeus turned himself into an eagle and raped her. She bore him three sons, one of whom was the king of Crete, Minos. She was the founder of the European race.

Leto

Leto was the mother of Artemis and Apollo. Zeus

made her pregnant, disguising both himself and Leto as quails. Hera found out and was jealous, and had Python, the serpent, pursue her. Leto gave birth to Artemis in Ortygia, and to Apollo on Delos, between a date-palm and an olive-tree.

> 'The mother is the pivot around which the home circle turns. If she finds that outside interests are tending to overshadow those of the home she must take steps to prevent it or her whole circle will suffer.'
>
> Mary Macaulay,
> *The Art of Marriage*, Penguin, 1952

Freya

Freya, in Norse mythology, was the wife of Odin, and the mother of Thor and Balder. One day, Balder reported that he believed his life was under threat. Freya, fearing for him, went about the whole of creation, making everything – living or otherwise – swear that it would not harm him. However, Loki, a duplicitous god, went to Freya dressed as a woman, and Freya accidentally revealed that the mistletoe did not swear, because it looked too young to do so.

Loki gave a mistletoe dart to a blind god, who was unable to join in with the new game of hurling missiles at Balder (who, of course, was untouched by them), and offered to guide his aim. The dart hit Balder, and he fell dead. The gods were all devastated, and Freya sent a messenger to the Underworld, to find out how Balder might live again. The messenger returned, saying that Balder might only come back if every living thing wept. Again, Freya told everything in creation to weep: according to Norse mythology, this is why condensation is found upon metals.

Great Mother

For ancient Welsh tribes, the Great Mother was the female element of creation. She was the goddess of fertility, the moon, summer, flowers, love, healing, seas, and water. The index finger was considered the 'mother finger', the most magical, which guided, beckoned, blessed and cursed.

The Birth of Hercules

Chief among the Greek gods, Zeus was somewhat less than the ideal husband and father. It was his habit to slip away to have his way with mortal women, disguised in the hope that his wife Hera would not notice. When Zeus decided to father the most renowned of Greek heroes, Hercules, he went to considerable lengths, bribing the sun not to appear for three days, and the moon to travel more slowly, so he could enjoy an extended night of passion with the mortal Alcmene, disguised as her absent husband.

During her pregnancy it was obvious she was carrying the baby of a god: he was enormous, and the birth was certain to be difficult. It was made doubly so by the interference of Zeus's jealous wife; she sent Eileithyia, the goddess invoked by pregnant women, to sit near her, cross-legged, with her fingers intertwined – powerful spells to prevent childbirth.

Alcmene was sure she would not survive the ordeal, but one of her servants, Galanthis, tricked the goddess by declaring that Hercules had been safely delivered. Eileithyia sprang up, breaking the spell, and the hero was born. Galanthis, for her deception, was turned into a weasel, and because she had lied to help a woman give birth – weasel words – she was condemned to bear her own young through her mouth. The Greeks and Romans evidently believed this was how weasels bore their young! Hercules, however, started as he meant to go on, strangling two snakes, sent by the jealous Hera, while still in his cradle.

Celluloid Mothers

Ten Films About Motherhood

Terms of Endearment
Steel Magnolias
Mother Didn't Tell Me
Mother Is A Freshman
Serial Mom
Mama
Throw Momma from the Train
Freaky Friday
Mother Knows Best
Mother Love

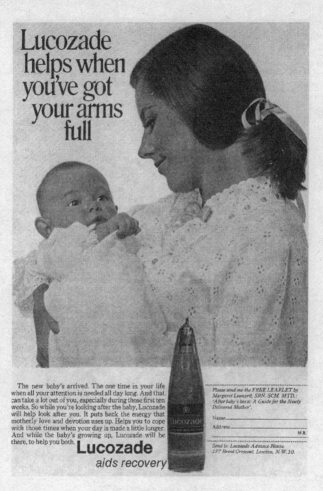

Lucozade targets new mums in 1972.

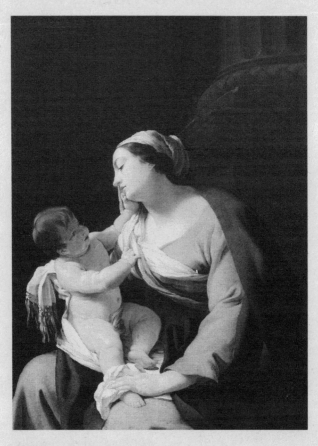

Virgin and Child, Simon Vouet, c. 1640; Ashmolean Museum, Oxford.

Thank you For Having Me

A History of Mothering Sunday

Not all of the ancient British traditions associated with motherhood have died out. One of them is still very much alive: Mother's Day, or Mothering Sunday.

Mother's Day and Mothering Sunday are actually two very different things, although they've merged together during the last century or so. Mothering Sunday has its origins way back in the Middle Ages, and the date on which it was celebrated was the fourth Sunday in Lent. The tradition wasn't actually connected with human mothers at all: on that day, everybody used to go to the main diocesan church, also called the 'Mother Church'. In the sixteenth century, the Reformation quashed many Catholic tendencies in England, and the emphasis on the 'Mother Church' was gradually replaced by the mother of the family.

> **'You cannot catch a child's spirit by running after it; you must stand still and for love it will soon itself return.'**
> Arthur Miller

In the seventeenth century, servants were allowed to return home on Mothering Sunday, and they usually gave little trinkets to their mothers as gifts, or presented them with a simnel cake. The tradition peaked during the Victorian era, when the mother was seen to be at the centre of all social structures, but the tradition fell into a decline after that.

The Americans started Mother's Day in the early twentieth century, when Anna Jarvis commemorated her mother's death in 1908, on the second Sunday in May. When the GIs came over to Britain during the Second World War, they revitalised the old British custom, to celebrate their absent mothers, adding their own festivities to the celebration of Mothering Sunday in March.

These days, over 25 million Mother's Day cards are sent in Britain every year. You can now look forward to receiving yours.

Copyright Notices

Text
p.6, 9, 39   Statistics from *Social Trends*, Office for National Statistics, © Crown Copyright 1998

Illustrations
p.3   *The Fugitive*, © RKO, 1947. Photograph courtesy of the Kobal Collection.
p.4   © Ladybird Books, 1958.
p.8   © Cow & Gate, 1971.
p.10 *Marriage is a Private Affair,* © MGM, 1944. Photograph courtesy of the Kobal Collection.
p.12 © Harvey Scruton, 1951.
p.15 © Ashmolean Museum, Oxford.
p.18 *The Lady is Willing*, © Columbia 1942. Photograph courtesy of the Kobal Collection.
p.21 © Oxo, 1986.
p.25 *Sparrows,* © Mary Pickford Company, 1926. Photograph courtesy of the Kobal Collection.
p.29 © Britvic, 1998.
p.37 © *Independent on Sunday*, 1998.
p.38 © Johnson & Johnson, 1957.
p.42 Photograph courtesy of the Kobal Collection.
p.46 © SmithKline Beecham, 1972.
p.48 © Ashmolean Museum, Oxford.

Purple House Limited has done its best to acknowledge the authors of all quotations and illustrations used in this book, but has not been able to make contact with everyone whose work is featured. If your work has not been acknowledged, please contact Purple House Limited, who will be happy to make proper acknowledgement if this book is reprinted or reissued.